Fitness for Busy Professionals

The Busy Professional's Guide to Fitness

Hina Victor

Fitness for Busy Professionals
Copyright © 2023 by Hina Victor

Printed in Pakistan by Hina

Dedication

This book is devoted to you. I know how hard it tends to be to shuffle a requesting position, family obligations, and individual responsibilities while as yet carving out opportunity to focus on your wellbeing and wellness. Yet, I additionally know that with the right methodologies and mentality, it's feasible to accomplish your wellness objectives and further develop your general prosperity.

I composed this book in light of occupied experts, offering down to earth tips and guidance for fitting in practice and sound propensities in any event, when your timetable is pressed. My expectation is that this book will act as a wellspring of motivation and inspiration for you on your wellness process, and that it will assist you with understanding that regardless of how occupied you will be, you can in any case set aside a few minutes for your wellbeing.

Much thanks to you for getting some margin to peruse this book, and for putting resources into yourself and your wellbeing. Here are to a morejoyful,betteryou.

Hina Victor

Table of Contents

Foreword

As a bustling proficient myself, I know how hard it very well may be to set aside a few minutes for wellness and exercise. Yet, I additionally know that focusing on our wellbeing and prosperity, particularly in the present quick moving and upsetting world is so significant. That is the reason I'm excited to present this book on "Readiness for Occupied Experts."

In this book, you'll track down reasonable tips and methodologies for integrating exercise and solid propensities into your bustling timetable. From time-productive exercises to quality dinner arranging, the creator offers bits of knowledge and guidance in view of long stretches of involvement working with occupied experts such as you.

What I value most about this book is the writer's way to deal with wellness. Instead of upholding for severe weight control plans or outrageous activity regimens, she stresses the significance of finding what works for you and making maintainable way of life changes. This is key for occupied experts who need to adjust work, family, and individual responsibilities while as yet setting aside a few minutes for their wellbeing.

Whether you're a bustling chief, business visionary or working guardian, this book brings something to the table. I urge you to understand it, evaluate the tips and techniques, and perceive how they can assist you with accomplishing your wellness objectives and further develop your general prosperity.

Much thanks to you to the creator for sharing her skill and experiences, and to every one of the bustling experts out there who are focusing on their wellbeing.

Hina Victor

Preface

As a wellness proficient and occupied business visionary myself, I know how hard it tends to be to adjust work, family, and individual responsibilities while as yet setting aside a few minutes for practice and sound propensities. However, I likewise know that it's feasible to accomplish your wellness objectives, in any event, when you have a pressed timetable.

That is the reason I composed this book on "Qualification for Occupied Experts." In these pages, you'll find viable tips and procedures for fitting in practice and solid propensities, regardless of how occupied you are. From speedy and compelling exercises to straightforward dinner arranging tips, this book is intended to assist you with making feasible way of life changes that will work on your wellbeing and prosperity over the long haul.

However, this book isn't just about wellness. It's tied in with tracking down balance in a bustling world, and dealing with yourself amidst every one of the requests and tensions of current life. It's tied in with perceiving that our wellbeing is our most important resource, and that we can't bear to disregard it, regardless of how occupied we are.

I've composed this book considering occupied experts, since I realize firsthand the way that difficult it very well may be to set aside a few minutes for wellness in a rushed timetable. Yet, I likewise know that with the right attitude and procedures, it's feasible to accomplish your wellness objectives and further develop your general prosperity.

So assuming you're a bustling proficient hoping to focus on your wellbeing and wellness, I welcome you to plunge into this book and find the methodologies and bits of knowledge that have assisted endless others with preferring you. Here are to a more joyful, better you.

Hina Victor

Introduction

Do you battle to set aside opportunity for practice and solid propensities? Do you feel like your bustling timetable is keeping you away from accomplishing your wellness objectives? Assuming this is the case, you're in good company. As a wellness proficient and occupied business visionary myself, I realize how testing it tends to be to adjust work, family, and individual responsibilities while as yet focusing on our wellbeing and prosperity.

Yet, here's the uplifting news: accomplishing your wellness objectives, in any event, when you're busy is conceivable. As a matter of fact, I accept that wellness can be the establishment for outcome in all everyday issues. At the point when we deal with our bodies, we have more energy, concentration, and strength to handle the difficulties of work and life.

That is the reason I composed this book on "Qualification for Occupied Experts." In these pages, you'll find functional tips and methodologies for fitting in practice and solid propensities, regardless of how occupied you are. Whether you're a bustling leader, business person, or working guardian, this book is intended to assist you with making economical way of life changes that will work on your wellbeing and prosperity over the long haul.

Yet, this book isn't just about wellness. It's tied in with tracking down balance in a bustling world, and dealing with ourselves amidst every one of the requests and tensions of present day life.

It's tied in with perceiving that our wellbeing is our most important resource, and that we can't bear to disregard it, regardless of how occupied we are.

So on the off chance that you're prepared to focus on your wellbeing and wellness, even amidst a bustling timetable, I welcome you to plunge into this book and find the techniques and experiences that have assisted endless others with preferring you. Here are to a more joyful, better you.

Hina Victor

Chapter 1:
The Bustling Proficient's Manual for Wellness

As a bustling proficient, you realize that time is your most significant resource. Adjusting work, family, and individual responsibilities can be a test, and setting our wellbeing and wellness aside for later is simple. However, here's reality: ignoring our wellbeing and wellness can really make us less viable in all everyday issues. At the point when we focus on our wellbeing, we have more energy, concentration, and flexibility to handle the difficulties of work and life.

In this part, we'll investigate methodologies for fitting in practice and sound propensities, regardless of how occupied you are. From defining sensible objectives to capitalizing on your time, these tips and experiences will assist you with making an economical wellness schedule that works for your bustling way of life.

Putting forth Practical Objectives

The initial step to accomplishing any objective is to set reasonable assumptions. With regards to wellness, this implies recognizing that you might not have as much time as you might want to give to practice and sound propensities. In any case, that doesn't mean you can't gain ground. By putting forth practical objectives and zeroing in on little, reachable advances, you can make a wellness schedule that squeezes into your bustling timetable.

One powerful methodology is to break your wellness objectives into more modest, more reasonable advances. For instance, in the event that you want to shed 10 pounds, you could begin by zeroing in on losing one pound each week. This could mean rolling out little improvements to your eating routine, like removing sweet beverages or nibbling on products of the soil rather than chips. After some time, these little changes can amount to critical advancement.

Taking full advantage of Your Time

At the point when you're occupied, consistently counts. That is the reason it's critical to take advantage of your opportunity with regards to wellness. This could mean exploiting brief breaks during the day to do a speedy exercise, or planning your exercises for times when you're probably going to stay with them.

One powerful methodology is to integrate practice into your everyday daily schedule. For instance, you could have a go at trekking or strolling to work as opposed to driving, or using the stairwell rather than the lift. You could likewise consider integrating exercise into your mid-day break, for example, by doing a fast yoga normal or going for an energetic stroll outside.

Tracking down Responsibility and Backing

Remaining spurred and responsible is vital to staying with any wellness schedule. At the point when you're occupied, it very well may be not difficult to rationalize or neglect your wellness objectives. However, by finding responsibility and backing, you can remain focused and gain ground in any event, when life gets furious.

One successful technique is to find an exercise mate or responsibility accomplice. This may be a collaborator or companion who shares your wellness objectives, or somebody you meet through a wellness class or online local area. By checking in with one another consistently and supporting each other's advancement, you can remain spurred and responsible.

End

Accomplishing your wellness objectives as a bustling proficient is conceivable; however it requires a touch of imagination, arranging, and perseverance. By defining sensible objectives, capitalizing on your time, and finding responsibility and backing, you can make a practical wellness schedule that squeezes into your bustling way of life. In the following section, we'll investigate fast and successful exercises that can assist you with fitting in work-out even on the most active of days.

Chapter 2:
Fit in Five

At the point when you're in the middle of, carving out opportunity for exercise can be a test. In any case, regardless of whether you just have five minutes in excess, you can in any case get in a speedy, successful exercise that will assist you with feeling empowered and centered. In this section, we'll investigate a few five-minute exercises that you can do anyplace, whenever, with next to no gear. These exercises are intended to work your whole body and get your pulse up, so you can take full advantage of your time and feel incredible the entire day.

The Five-Minute Bodyweight Circuit

This exercise is intended to work your whole body and get your pulse up in only five minutes. Play out each activity for 30 seconds, with 10 seconds of in the middle between. Rehash the circuit multiple times for a sum of five minutes.

Hopping Jacks: Stand with your feet together and your arms at your sides. Hop your feet out to the sides and raise your arms above. Bounce your feet back together and bring down your arms to your sides. Rehash for 30 seconds.

Push-Ups: Begin in a board position with your hands shoulder-width separated and your feet together. Lower your body to the cold earth, keeping your elbows near your sides. Push back up to the beginning position. Rehash for 30 seconds.

Squats: Stand with your feet shoulder-width separated and your arms at your sides. Twist your knees and lower your body down as though you were sitting in a seat. Stand back up to the beginning position. Rehash for 30 seconds.

Hikers: Begin in a board position with your hands shoulder-width separated and your feet together. Bring your right knee up to your chest, then, at that point, immediately switch legs, bringing your surrendered knee to your chest. Rehash for 30 seconds.

Burgees: Begin in a standing position. Twist down and put your hands on the ground. Bounce your feet back into a board position, then, at that point, immediately hop them back up to your hands. Stand up and bounce, arriving at your arms above. Rehash for 30 seconds.

The Five-Minute Cardio Impact

This exercise is intended to get your pulse up and consume calories in only five minutes. Play out each activity for 30 seconds, with 10 seconds of in the middle between. Rehash the circuit multiple times for a sum of five minutes.

Hopping Jacks: Stand with your feet together and your arms at your sides. Hop your feet out to the sides and raise your arms above. Bounce your feet back together and bring down your arms to your sides. Rehash for 30 seconds.

High Knees: Stand with your feet hip-width separated. Lift one knee up to your chest, then, at that point, immediately switch legs, lifting your other knee up to your chest. Keep exchanging legs as fast as workable for 30 seconds.

Butt Kicks: Stand with your feet hip-width separated. Kick one heel up to your posterior, then, at that point, immediately switch legs, kicking your other heel up to your rear end. Keep substituting legs as fast as feasible for 30 seconds.

Bounce Squats: Stand with your feet shoulder-width separated. Twist your knees and lower your body down as though you were sitting in a seat. Bounce up as high as possible, then land delicately and promptly lower down into a squat. Rehash for 30 seconds.

Stop and go aerobic exercise (HIIT): Pick any extreme focus work out, for example, running, bouncing

Chapter 3:
The Wellbeing Diagram

Being solid and fit isn't just about working out and eating right; it's additionally about dealing with your psychological and close to home prosperity. In this section, we'll investigate the idea of a wellbeing diagram, an arrangement that frames the techniques you can use to accomplish ideal wellbeing in all parts of your life. By making your own wellbeing outline, you'll have the option to focus on your wellbeing and prosperity, prompting a more joyful, better life.

Surveying Your Present status of Wellbeing

Before you can make your wellbeing diagram, evaluating your present status of wellness is significant. Find opportunity to ponder your physical, mental, and profound wellbeing. What regions would you say you are now doing great ready? Where do you have to get to the next level? Utilize the accompanying inquiries to direct your appearance:

Actual Wellbeing:

Do you get sufficient activity every week?
Do you eat a fair, nutritious eating routine?
Do you get sufficient rest every evening?
Do you have any persistent medical issue that require consideration?
Emotional wellness:

Do you have an emotionally supportive network that you can go to in the midst of hardship?
Do you oversee pressure actually?
Do you participate in exercises that give you pleasure and satisfaction?

Do you have an inspirational perspective on life?
Profound Wellbeing:

Do you have solid associations with loved ones?
Do you feel genuinely satisfied in your work or leisure activities?
Do you have a feeling of direction or importance in your life?
Do you get some margin for taking care of oneself and self-reflection?
Making Your Wellbeing Plan

Whenever you've evaluated your present status of wellbeing now is the right time to make your health outline. This plan ought to be custom-made to your singular requirements and objectives, and ought to consider your present status of wellbeing. Here are moves toward follow while making your health outline:

Put forth Objectives: Ponder what you need to accomplish as far as your physical, mental, and close to home wellbeing. Set explicit, quantifiable objectives that are reasonable and feasible.

Recognize Methodologies: Distinguish the systems that you will use to accomplish your objectives. These may incorporate things like working out routinely, eating a solid eating regimen, thinking, or rehearsing taking care of oneself.

Make an Arrangement: Make an arrangement for how you will execute these systems into your day to day routine. This might include booking exercises, dinner preparing, or carving out opportunity every day for taking care of oneself.

Assess Your Advancement: Consistently assess your advancement and change your arrangement on a case by case basis. This will assist you with remaining focused and keep gaining ground towards your objectives.

By following these means, you can make a wellbeing plan that will assist you with accomplishing ideal wellbeing in all parts of your life. Make sure to focus on taking care of oneself and self-reflection, and feel free to request help or backing when required. With a strong wellbeing plan set up, you can have a more joyful, better existence.

Chapter 4:
The Psyche Body Association

The association between our psyches and bodies is a strong one, and can fundamentally affect our general wellbeing and prosperity. In this section, we'll investigate the idea of the psyche body association and how it very well may be utilized to work on our physical, mental, and profound wellbeing.

Understanding the Psyche Body Association

The psyche body association alludes to the possibility that our psychological and profound states can influence our actual wellbeing as well as the other way around. For instance, persistent pressure or nervousness can prompt actual side effects like cerebral pains, muscle strain, and stomach related issues. Likewise, actual diseases, for example, constant torment or sickness can altogether affect our psychological and close to home prosperity.

The psyche body association can likewise be utilized to work on our wellbeing. By rehearsing strategies that advance unwinding and diminish pressure, like contemplation, yoga, or profound breathing, we can work on our actual wellbeing and lessen our gamble of constant ailment.

Rehearsing Psyche Body Methods

There are an assortment of psyche body methods that can be utilized to work on our general wellbeing and prosperity. Here are a few models:

Contemplation: Reflection includes concentrating on a particular item, thought, or movement, and can assist with diminishing pressure and tension, further develop rest, and increment sensations of prosperity.

Yoga: Yoga includes a progression of stances and breathing procedures that advance unwinding and lessen pressure. It can likewise further develop adaptability, strength, and equilibrium.

Jujitsu: Judo is a delicate type of activity that includes slow, streaming developments and profound relaxing. It can further develop equilibrium, adaptability, and diminish pressure and uneasiness.

Profound Relaxing: Profound breathing activities include taking sluggish, full breaths, which can assist with lessening pressure and nervousness, further develop concentration and fixation, and increment sensations of unwinding.

Integrating Psyche Body Procedures into Your Everyday Daily schedule

To receive the rewards of the psyche body association, integrating these procedures into your day to day routine is significant. Here are a few ways to get everything rolling:

Begin Little: Start with only a couple of moments of reflection or profound breathing every day, and continuously increment how much time as you become more agreeable.

Practice Reliably: Consistency is key with regards to mind-body procedures. Put away a particular time every day to practice, and stick to it.

Find What Works for You: Everybody's inclinations and necessities are different with regards to mind-body procedures. Try different things with various practices to find what turns out best for you.

By integrating mind-body procedures into your everyday daily schedule, you can work on your physical, mental, and profound wellbeing, and accomplish a more noteworthy feeling of prosperity. Keep in mind, the brain and body are interconnected, and dealing with both is fundamental for ideal wellbeing..

Chapter 5:
The 15-Minute Exercise

As a bustling proficient, carving out opportunity to exercise can be a test. Yet, with a 15-minute exercise, you can fit in a fast and viable gym routine even on your most active days. In this part, we'll investigate the advantages of a 15-minute exercise and give an example exercise routine everyday practice to kick you off.

Advantages of a 15-Minute Exercise

A 15-minute exercise can give different advantages, including:

Time-productive: With only 15 minutes, you can fit in a speedy exercise without forfeiting a lot of your bustling timetable.

Expanded energy: A short exercise can assist with supporting your energy levels and work on your state of mind.

Worked on cardiovascular wellbeing a 15-minute exercise can be intended to get your pulse up, which can work on your cardiovascular wellbeing.

Strength working: With the right activities, you can likewise develop fortitude during a 15-minute exercise.

Test 15-Minute Exercise routine Daily practice

Here is an example 15-minute gym routine schedule that should be possible at home or in the workplace:

Warm-up: Start with a five-minute warm-up, which can remember running for place, bouncing jacks, or extending.

Squats: Begin with 30 seconds of squats, zeroing in on legitimate structure and keeping your weight in your heels.

Push-ups: Do 10 push-ups, either on your toes or kneeling down, zeroing in on keeping your center locked in.

Rushes: Complete 30 seconds of lurches, exchanging legs with every redundancy.

Board: Hold a board for 30 seconds, zeroing in on keeping your center connected with and keeping up with legitimate structure.

Hopping jacks: Finish the exercise with 30 seconds of bouncing jacks to get your pulse up.

Cool-Down

Finish the exercise with a five-minute cool-down, which can incorporate extending or a sluggish stroll to bring your pulse down.

Tweaking Your 15-Minute Exercise

The example exercise above is only one illustration of a 15-minute exercise routine daily schedule. You can alter your exercise in view of your wellness level, inclinations, and objectives. A few different activities that can be integrated into a 15-minute exercise include:

Burgees
High knees
Hikers
Rear arm muscle plunges
Leg lifts
Bicep twists
End

A 15-minute exercise is an incredible method for squeezing exercise into your bustling timetable. With a short however powerful everyday practice, you can receive the rewards of worked on actual wellness and expanded energy. Make sure to continuously zero in on legitimate structure and to pay attention to your body to forestall injury.

Chapter 6:
Fuel Your Body, Fuel Your Prosperity

As a bustling proficient, you realize that your body and brain need fuel to perform at their best. In this part, we'll investigate the significance of legitimate sustenance and give tips to energizing your body for progress.

Why Legitimate Sustenance Matters

The food you eat gives the structure blocks to your body and cerebrum to work. Eating a reasonable eating routine that incorporates different supplement thick food sources can give a scope of advantages, including:

Expanded energy: Eating nutritious food sources can give the energy you want to muscle through your bustling days.

Worked on mental lucidity certain food sources can further develop mind capability, including memory and concentration

Helped invulnerable framework: Appropriate nourishment can assist with supporting your insusceptible framework, decreasing your gamble of ailment.

Kept up with weight a fair eating routine can assist you with keeping a sound weight, diminishing your gamble of persistent sicknesses like coronary illness and diabetes.

Ways to fuel Your Body for Progress

Prepare: Take time toward the start of the week to design out your feasts and tidbits. This can assist you with trying not to snatch unfortunate choices when you're in a rush.

Consolidate protein: Protein is significant for building and fixing tissues in your body. Try to remember a wellspring of protein for every feast and bite.

Pick supplement thick food sources: Rather than topping off on void calories, decide on food sources that are loaded with supplements like natural products, vegetables, entire grains, and lean proteins.

Remain hydrated: Drinking sufficient water is significant for generally speaking wellbeing, and can likewise assist you with keeping up with energy levels and concentration.

Limit handled food varieties: Handled food varieties are many times high in sodium, sugar, and undesirable fats. Limit your admission and select entire, natural food varieties all things being equal.

Test Feast Plan

Here is an example feast plan for a bustling proficient:

Breakfast: Greek yogurt with new berries and a sprinkle of granola

Nibble: Apple cuts with almond spread

Lunch: Barbecued chicken plate of mixed greens with blended greens, veggies, and a balsamic vinaigrette

Nibble: Hard-bubbled egg and carrot sticks

Supper: Barbecued salmon with simmered vegetables and quinoa

End

Legitimate sustenance is a fundamental part of a sound way of life, and can assume a vital part in your prosperity as a bustling proficient. By integrating supplement thick food varieties and preparing, you can fuel your body for progress and accomplish your objectives. Make sure to pay attention to your body and make changes depending on the situation to find the sustenance plan that turns out best for you.

Chapter 7:

From Work area to Exercise center

As a bustling proficient, carving out opportunity to exercise can be a test. In any case, with a touch of arranging and imagination, you can fit in a gym routine even on your most active days. In this section, we'll share ways to go from work area to exercise center and capitalizing on your restricted time.

Prepare

The way to fitting in an exercise is to prepare. Take a gander at your timetable for the week and figure out pockets of opportunity when you can crush in a speedy exercise. You might have to get up somewhat prior, avoid your mid-day break, or exercise after work, however with some inventive reasoning, you can carve out the opportunity.

Gather Your Pack

Make it simple to go from work to the red center by gathering your pack ahead of time. Incorporate all that you'll require for your exercise, for example, exercise garments, tennis shoes, a water bottle, and any gear you intend to utilize.

Utilize Your Mid-day Break

In the event that you can't set aside opportunity previously or after work to work out considers utilizing your mid-day break Search for a red center or wellness studio close to your office, or set out outside toward a run or walk. You can likewise do a speedy exercise in your office or a close by park.

Perform multiple tasks

Utilize your exercise time to get up to speed with work errands or calls. Carry your PC or telephone to the red center and work while you're on the treadmill or bicycle. Simply make certain to zero in on your structure and wellbeing first.

Take full advantage of Your Exercise
At the point when you're in a rush, it's critical to capitalize on your exercise. Pick focused energy exercises that will get your pulse up and consume calories rapidly. Stretch preparation, high-intensity aerobics, and HIIT exercises are extraordinary choices.

Test Exercise

Here is an example exercise that you can do in a short time or less:

Warm-up: 5 minutes on the treadmill or circular machine

Circuit 1: Complete each activity for 1 moment, rest for 30 seconds after each activity.

Squat leaps
Push-ups
Board jacks
Hand weight lines
Circuit 2: Complete each activity for 1 moment, rest for 30 seconds after each activity.

Burgees
Hikers
Russian turns
Bicep twists
Cool-down: 5 minutes of extending

End

With just enough preparation and imagination, you can fit in a gym routine even on your most active days. Utilize your mid-day break, perform multiple tasks, and take advantage of your exercise time to accomplish your wellness objectives. Make sure to pay attention to your body and make changes on a case by case basis to find the activity plan that turns out best for you.

Chapter 8: Past Burnout

As a bustling proficient, it's not difficult to become overpowered and worn out. At the point when you're continually shuffling work, family, and different obligations, it can feel like time is running out for taking care of oneself. Be that as it may, dealing with you is fundamental for forestalling burnout and keeping a solid balance between serious and fun activities. In this part, we'll investigate the significance of taking care of oneself and give tips to moving past burnout.

Perceive the Indications of Burnout
The most important phase in forestalling burnout perceives the signs. Burnout can appear in various ways, including actual depletion, profound weariness, skepticism, and diminished efficiency. In the event that you're encountering any of these side effects, it's essential to make a move before burnout turns into a constant issue.

Focus on Taking care of one
Taking care of oneself is fundamental for forestalling burnout and keeping a sound balance between serious and fun activities. This incorporates requiring some investment for work out, good dieting, unwinding, and social association. Make taking care of oneself a non-debatable piece of your daily schedule, very much like some other significant undertaking.

Put down stopping points
One of the greatest supporters of burnout is an absence of limits. Figure out how to express no to responsibilities that don't line up with your objectives or values, and set sensible assumptions for you and others. Convey your limits plainly, and stick to them.

Practice Care

Care is an integral asset for overseeing pressure and forestalling burnout. Take time every day to rehearse care reflection, profound breathing, or other unwinding procedures. These practices can assist you with remaining present and zeroed in, even amidst a feverish working day.

Look for Help

At last, make sure to look for help when you want it. This might incorporate conversing with a companion or relative, looking for proficient directing, or joining a care group. Anything type of help you pick, recollect that you don't need to go through burnout alone.

End

Burnout is a typical issue among occupied experts, yet it doesn't need to be unavoidable. By perceiving the indications of burnout, focusing on taking care of one, defining limits, rehearsing care, and looking for help, you can move past burnout and accomplish a better balance between fun and serious activities. Keep in mind, dealing with yourself is fundamental for keeping up with your physical and mental prosperity, and for being the best version of yourself in all parts of your life.

Chapter 9:
The Wellness Attitude

Wellness isn't just about actual strength and perseverance. It's likewise about mental strength and versatility. In this part, we'll investigate the significance of fostering a wellness outlook and give tips to developing mental strength.

Embrace the Interaction
Wellness is an excursion, not an objective. It's vital to embrace the cycle and spotlight on progress, as opposed flawlessly. Celebrate little triumphs en route, and don't get deterred by difficulties or levels.

Put forth Practical Objectives
Laying out objectives is significant for remaining propelled and zeroed in, however it's essential to define practical objectives that line up with your abilities to ongoing and way of life. Make an arrangement that is testing however reachable, and separate your objectives into more modest, more sensible advances.

Practice Self-Empathy
Self-empathy is fundamental for keeping an inspirational perspective and staying balanced. Indulge yourself with the very consideration and understanding that you would offer a dear companion. Try not to whip yourself over mix-ups or misfortunes; all things being equal, use them as learning open doors

Challenge Your Cutoff points
To foster mental sturdiness, you really want to challenge your cutoff points. Propel yourself out of your usual range of familiarity and attempt new things. Whether it's another work-out daily practice, another wellness challenge, or another side interest,

venturing beyond your usual range of familiarity can assist you with building flexibility and certainty.

Remain Positive

Keeping an uplifting outlook is vital to developing a wellness mentality. Center around the headway you've made, instead of the impediments ahead. Encircle yourself with positive individuals who support your objectives and offer your qualities. Also, above all, be caring to yourself.

End

Fostering a wellness mentality is fundamental for making long haul progress and keeping a sound way of life. By embracing the cycle, putting forth reasonable objectives, rehearsing self-empathy, testing your cutoff points, and remaining positive, you can develop the psychological sturdiness you really want to conquer hindrances and accomplish your wellness objectives. Keep in mind, wellness isn't just about actual strength and perseverance; it's additionally about mental strength and flexibility.

Chapter 10:
Fit forever

Wellness isn't simply a transitory objective or a convenient solution. A long lasting pursuit can significantly affect your general wellbeing and prosperity. In this section, we'll investigate the idea of being "fit forever" and give tips to keeping a solid way of life in the long haul.

Find Exercises You Appreciate

One of the keys to remaining fit for life is finding proactive tasks that you appreciate. Whether it's climbing, trekking, swimming, moving, or playing sports, integrating exercises that you really appreciate into your everyday schedule can assist with making wellness a characteristic piece of your life.

Regularly practice Solid Decisions

Making sound propensities is critical for keeping a solid way of life. Pick supplement thick food varieties, remain hydrated, and go for the gold every evening. Integrating these solid propensities into your everyday schedule can assist with guaranteeing that you're dealing with your body in the long haul.

Focus on Rest and Recuperation

Rest and recuperation are similarly essentially as significant as actual work with regards to keeping a solid way of life. Allow yourself to take rest days and focus on recuperation exercises like extending, froth rolling, and yoga. This will help forestall burnout and injury, and keep you feeling stimulated and spurred.

Remain Responsible

Responsibility is key with regards to keeping a solid way of life. Find an exercise accomplice, join a wellness local area, or recruit a fitness coach or mentor. Having somebody to consider you responsible can assist with keeping you on target and inspired.

Continue To challenge yourself

Remaining fit for life implies proceeding to challenge yourself truly and intellectually. Put forth new objectives, attempt new exercises, and propel yourself out of your usual range of familiarity. This will assist you with remaining drew in and roused, and guarantee that you keep on seeing improvement over the long haul.

End

Being good for life implies committing to your wellbeing and prosperity that endures forever. By finding exercises you appreciate, practicing solid decisions all the time, focusing on rest and recuperation, remaining responsible, and testing yourself, you can keep a sound way of life that upholds you're drawn out objectives. Keep in mind, wellness isn't just about actual strength and perseverance; it's likewise about mental strength and flexibility, and the capacity to keep going with solid decisions for a lifetime.